101 CARDIO WORKOUTS

Created by Dominique & Erik Myers

ISBN: 9798264247972

Before you start this exercise program or make any changes in your lifestyle you must get your doctor or physician's approval. This product is for informational purposes only and is not meant as medical advice, nor is it a substitute for medical advice. In no way will Dominique or Erik Myers be held responsible for any injuries or problems that may occur due to the use of this program or advice contained within. Consult with a doctor before starting any exercise program. Performing exercise of all types can pose a risk to the exerciser. Before exercising make certain that the equipment is in good condition and be sure to know your own physical limits. Adequate warm up and cool downs should be undertaken before and after any exercise. If you experience any pain, discomfort, dizziness or shortness of breath, stop exercising immediately and consult your doctor. Please understand that you are solely responsible for the way information from this book by Dominique and Erik Myers is perceived and utilized and you do so at your own risk.

No time? No problem. With *101 Cardio Workouts*, you'll discover a powerful collection of quick, high-intensity workouts designed to deliver maximum results in minimum time. This is perfect for busy professionals, parents, athletes, or anyone who wants to torch calories, improve their cardio, and feel stronger—without spending hours in the gym.

Inside, you'll find:

✓**101 unique cardio workouts** — no two are the same, keeping your training fresh and exciting.
✓ **Bodyweight-only options** — so you can train anywhere, anytime.
✓ **Fat-burning cardio circuits** — proven to skyrocket your metabolism.
✓ **Strength and core routines** — sculpt lean muscle and build total-body power.
✓ **Scalable for all fitness levels** — whether you're a beginner or advanced athlete.
✓ **Minimal equipment variations** — dumbbells, bands, or just your body.

Each workout is designed to last just 20 minutes, making it easy to stay consistent—even on your busiest days. Whether your goal is weight loss, muscle tone, or improved athletic performance, this book gives you the blueprint to transform your body and energy levels.

Stop making excuses. Start making progress.
Your fittest self is only 20 minutes away.

WORKOUT 1

1. Warm-up: 1 minute of Dynamic Lunges
2. Circuit: Perform 40s work / 20s rest per exercise
- Lunges
- Plank
- Jump Rope
- Jump Squats
- Flutter Kicks
3. Repeat circuit for 3 rounds (about 15 minutes total)
4. Cool-down: 2 minutes of Hamstring Stretch

Tip: Increase difficulty by adding weights, explosive movements, or reducing rest time.

WORKOUT 2:

1. Warm-up: 1 minute of Butt Kicks
2. Circuit: Perform 20s work / 10s rest per exercise
- Plank
- Toe Touches
- High Knees
- Skater Jumps
- Squats
3. Repeat circuit for 6 rounds (about 15 minutes total)
4. Cool-down: 2 minutes of Cat-Cow Stretch

Tip: Increase difficulty by adding weights, explosive movements, or reducing rest time.

WORKOUT 3:

1. Warm-up: 1 minute of Arm Circles
2. Circuit: Perform 40s work / 20s rest per exercise
- Calf Raises
- Bicycle Crunches
- Flutter Kicks
- V-Ups
- Push-ups
3. Repeat circuit for 3 rounds (about 15 minutes total)
4. Cool-down: 2 minutes of Downward Dog

Tip: Increase difficulty by adding weights, explosive movements, or reducing rest time.

WORKOUT 4:

1. Warm-up: 1 minute of inchworms
2. Circuit: Perform 20s work / 10s rest per exercise
- Lunges
- Tricep Dips
- Bird Dogs
- Plank
- Leg Raises
3. Repeat circuit for 6 rounds (about 15 minutes total)
4. Cool-down: 2 minutes of Forward Fold Stretch

Tip: Increase difficulty by adding weights, explosive movements, or reducing rest time.

WORKOUT 5:

1. Warm-up: 1 minute of Jog in Place
2. Circuit: Perform 40s work / 20s rest per exercise
- Flutter Kicks
- Star Jumps
- Russian Twists
- Calf Raises
- High Knees
3. Repeat circuit for 3 rounds (about 15 minutes total)
4. Cool-down: 2 minutes of alternating quad stretch

Tip: Increase difficulty by adding weights, explosive movements, or reducing rest time.

WORKOUT 6:

1. Warm-up: 1 minute of Jumping Jacks
2. Circuit: Perform 20s work / 10s rest per exercise
- Star Jumps
- Tricep Dips
- Side Plank
- Flutter Kicks
- Plank
3. Repeat circuit for 6 rounds (about 15 minutes total)
4. Cool-down: 2 minutes of Cat-Cow Stretch

Tip: Increase difficulty by adding weights, explosive movements, or reducing rest time.

WORKOUT 7:

1. Warm-up: 1 minute of Side Shuffles
2. Circuit: Perform 40s work / 20s rest per exercise
- Push-ups
- Mountain Climbers
- V-Ups
- Jump Squats
- Lateral Bounds
3. Repeat circuit for 3 rounds (about 15 minutes total)
4. Cool-down: 2 minutes of Hamstring Stretch

Tip: Increase difficulty by adding weights, explosive movements, or reducing rest time.

WORKOUT 8:

1. Warm-up: 1 minute of inchworms
2. Circuit: Perform 20s work / 10s rest per exercise
- Bird Dogs
- Skater Jumps
- Squats
- Toe Touches
- Jumping Lunges
3. Repeat circuit for 6 rounds (about 15 minutes total)
4. Cool-down: 2 minutes of Child's Pose

Tip: Increase difficulty by adding weights, explosive movements, or reducing rest time.

WORKOUT 9:

1. Warm-up: 1 minute of Side Shuffles
2. Circuit: Perform 40s work / 20s rest per exercise
- High Knees
- Squats
- Bird Dogs
- Sumo Squats
- Leg Raises
3. Repeat circuit for 3 rounds (about 15 minutes total)
4. Cool-down: 2 minutes of Seated Twist

Tip: Increase difficulty by adding weights, explosive movements, or reducing rest time.

WORKOUT 10:

1. Warm-up: 1 minute of Dynamic Lunges
2. Circuit: Perform 20s work / 10s rest per exercise
- Bicycle Crunches
- Calf Raises
- V-Ups
- Dead Bugs
- Side Plank
3. Repeat circuit for 6 rounds (about 15 minutes total)
4. Cool-down: 2 minutes of Hip Flexor Stretch

Tip: Increase difficulty by adding weights, explosive movements, or reducing rest time.

WORKOUT 11:

1. Warm-up: 1 minute of inchworms
2. Circuit: Perform 40s work / 20s rest per exercise
- Bird Dogs
- Sprint in Place
- Flutter Kicks
- Squats
- Burpees
3. Repeat circuit for 3 rounds (about 15 minutes total)
4. Cool-down: 2 minutes of alternating quad stretch

Tip: Increase difficulty by adding weights, explosive movements, or reducing rest time.

WORKOUT 12:

1. Warm-up: 1 minute of Shadow Boxing
2. Circuit: Perform 20s work / 10s rest per exercise
- Flutter Kicks
- Dead Bugs
- Skater Jumps
- Burpees
- V-Ups
3. Repeat circuit for 6 rounds (about 15 minutes total)
4. Cool-down: 2 minutes of Forward Fold Stretch

Tip: Increase difficulty by adding weights, explosive movements, or reducing rest time.

WORKOUT 13:

1. Warm-up: 1 minute of Butt Kicks
2. Circuit: Perform 40s work / 20s rest per exercise
- Toe Touches
- Star Jumps
- Hollow Hold
- Sprint in Place
- Jump Rope
3. Repeat circuit for 3 rounds (about 15 minutes total)
4. Cool-down: 2 minutes of Downward Dog

Tip: Increase difficulty by adding weights, explosive movements, or reducing rest time.

WORKOUT 14:

1. Warm-up: 1 minute of Arm Circles
2. Circuit: Perform 20s work / 10s rest per exercise
- Plank
- Star Jumps
- Lateral Bounds
- Squats
- Calf Raises
3. Repeat circuit for 6 rounds (about 15 minutes total)
4. Cool-down: 2 minutes of alternating quad stretch

Tip: Increase difficulty by adding weights, explosive movements, or reducing rest time.

WORKOUT 15:

1. Warm-up: 1 minute of inchworms
2. Circuit: Perform 40s work / 20s rest per exercise
- Leg Raises
- Push-ups
- Toe Touches
- Glute Bridges
- Step-Ups
3. Repeat circuit for 3 rounds (about 15 minutes total)
4. Cool-down: 2 minutes of Hamstring Stretch

Tip: Increase difficulty by adding weights, explosive movements, or reducing rest time.

WORKOUT 16:

1. Warm-up: 1 minute of Jog in Place
2. Circuit: Perform 20s work / 10s rest per exercise
- Leg Raises
- High Knees
- Single-Leg Deadlifts (bodyweight)
- Toe Touches
- Bicycle Crunches
3. Repeat circuit for 6 rounds (about 15 minutes total)
4. Cool-down: 2 minutes of Forward Fold Stretch

Tip: Increase difficulty by adding weights, explosive movements, or reducing rest time.

WORKOUT 17:

1. Warm-up: 1 minute of Dynamic Lunges
2. Circuit: Perform 40s work / 20s rest per exercise
- Squats
- Leg Raises
- Tricep Dips
- Toe Touches
- Pike Push-ups
3. Repeat circuit for 3 rounds (about 15 minutes total)
4. Cool-down: 2 minutes of Child's Pose

Tip: Increase difficulty by adding weights, explosive movements, or reducing rest time.

WORKOUT 18:

1. Warm-up: 1 minute of Jog in Place
2. Circuit: Perform 20s work / 10s rest per exercise
- Jumping Lunges
- High Knees
- Leg Raises
- Bicycle Crunches
- Frog Jumps
3. Repeat circuit for 6 rounds (about 15 minutes total)
4. Cool-down: 2 minutes of alternating quad stretch

Tip: Increase difficulty by adding weights, explosive movements, or reducing rest time.

WORKOUT 19:

1. Warm-up: 1 minute of Side Shuffles
2. Circuit: Perform 40s work / 20s rest per exercise
- Squats
- Pike Push-ups
- Flutter Kicks
- Star Jumps
- Lateral Bounds
3. Repeat circuit for 3 rounds (about 15 minutes total)
4. Cool-down: 2 minutes of Forward Fold Stretch

Tip: Increase difficulty by adding weights, explosive movements, or reducing rest time.

WORKOUT 20:

1. Warm-up: 1 minute of Arm Circles
2. Circuit: Perform 20s work / 10s rest per exercise
- Single-Leg Deadlifts (bodyweight)
- Lateral Bounds
- Leg Raises
- Burpees
- Jump Squats
3. Repeat circuit for 6 rounds (about 15 minutes total)
4. Cool-down: 2 minutes of Forward Fold Stretch

Tip: Increase difficulty by adding weights, explosive movements, or reducing rest time.

WORKOUT 21:

1. Warm-up: 1 minute of Butt Kicks
2. Circuit: Perform 40s work / 20s rest per exercise
- Flutter Kicks
- Lunges
- Step-Ups
- Toe Touches
- Jump Squats
3. Repeat circuit for 3 rounds (about 15 minutes total)
4. Cool-down: 2 minutes of Cat-Cow Stretch

Tip: Increase difficulty by adding weights, explosive movements, or reducing rest time.

WORKOUT 22:

1. Warm-up: 1 minute of Shadow Boxing
2. Circuit: Perform 20s work / 10s rest per exercise
- Frog Jumps
- Pike Push-ups
- Dead Bugs
- Glute Bridges
- Hollow Hold
3. Repeat circuit for 6 rounds (about 15 minutes total)
4. Cool-down: 2 minutes of Child's Pose

Tip: Increase difficulty by adding weights, explosive movements, or reducing rest time.

WORKOUT 23:

1. Warm-up: 1 minute of High Knees (low intensity)
2. Circuit: Perform 40s work / 20s rest per exercise
- Side Plank
- Bicycle Crunches
- Sprint in Place
- Leg Raises
- Lunges
3. Repeat circuit for 3 rounds (about 15 minutes total)
4. Cool-down: 2 minutes of Cat-Cow Stretch

Tip: Increase difficulty by adding weights, explosive movements, or reducing rest time.

WORKOUT 24:

1. Warm-up: 1 minute of Side Shuffles
2. Circuit: Perform 20s work / 10s rest per exercise
- Frog Jumps
- Squats
- Mountain Climbers (slow)
- Flutter Kicks
- V-Ups
3. Repeat circuit for 6 rounds (about 15 minutes total)
4. Cool-down: 2 minutes of Hip Flexor Stretch

Tip: Increase difficulty by adding weights, explosive movements, or reducing rest time.

WORKOUT 25:

1. Warm-up: 1 minute of inchworms
2. Circuit: Perform 40s work / 20s rest per exercise
- Pike Push-ups
- Bird Dogs
- Side Plank
- Squats
- Mountain Climbers (slow)
3. Repeat circuit for 3 rounds (about 15 minutes total)
4. Cool-down: 2 minutes of alternating quad stretch

Tip: Increase difficulty by adding weights, explosive movements, or reducing rest time.

WORKOUT 26:

1. Warm-up: 1 minute of Side Shuffles
2. Circuit: Perform 20s work / 10s rest per exercise
- Bird Dogs
- Single-Leg Deadlifts (bodyweight)
- Sumo Squats
- Lateral Bounds
- Mountain Climbers (slow)
3. Repeat circuit for 6 rounds (about 15 minutes total)
4. Cool-down: 2 minutes of Downward Dog

Tip: Increase difficulty by adding weights, explosive movements, or reducing rest time.

WORKOUT 27:

1. Warm-up: 1 minute of Butt Kicks
2. Circuit: Perform 40s work / 20s rest per exercise
- Flutter Kicks
- Dead Bugs
- Step-Ups
- Lunges
- Pike Push-ups
3. Repeat circuit for 3 rounds (about 15 minutes total)
4. Cool-down: 2 minutes of Forward Fold Stretch

Tip: Increase difficulty by adding weights, explosive movements, or reducing rest time.

WORKOUT 28:

1. Warm-up: 1 minute of Side Shuffles
2. Circuit: Perform 20s work / 10s rest per exercise
- Glute Bridges
- Tricep Dips
- Jumping Lunges
- Lunges
- Lateral Bounds
3. Repeat circuit for 6 rounds (about 15 minutes total)
4. Cool-down: 2 minutes of alternating quad stretch

Tip: Increase difficulty by adding weights, explosive movements, or reducing rest time.

WORKOUT 29:

1. Warm-up: 1 minute of High Knees (low intensity)
2. Circuit: Perform 40s work / 20s rest per exercise
- Step-Ups
- Frog Jumps
- Leg Raises
- Flutter Kicks
- Sumo Squats
3. Repeat circuit for 3 rounds (about 15 minutes total)
4. Cool-down: 2 minutes of alternating quad stretch

Tip: Increase difficulty by adding weights, explosive movements, or reducing rest time.

WORKOUT 30:

1. Warm-up: 1 minute of inchworms
2. Circuit: Perform 20s work / 10s rest per exercise
- Single-Leg Deadlifts (bodyweight)
- Calf Raises
- Mountain Climbers (slow)
- Flutter Kicks
- Lunges
3. Repeat circuit for 6 rounds (about 15 minutes total)
4. Cool-down: 2 minutes of alternating quad stretch

Tip: Increase difficulty by adding weights, explosive movements, or reducing rest time.

WORKOUT 31:

1. Warm-up: 1 minute of Jumping Jacks
2. Circuit: Perform 40s work / 20s rest per exercise
- Pike Push-ups
- Mountain Climbers
- Leg Raises
- Toe Touches
- Frog Jumps
3. Repeat circuit for 3 rounds (about 15 minutes total)
4. Cool-down: 2 minutes of Hamstring Stretch

Tip: Increase difficulty by adding weights, explosive movements, or reducing rest time.

WORKOUT 32:

1. Warm-up: 1 minute of Arm Circles
2. Circuit: Perform 20s work / 10s rest per exercise
- Sumo Squats
- Mountain Climbers (slow)
- Jump Rope
- Jump Squats
- Lateral Bounds
3. Repeat circuit for 6 rounds (about 15 minutes total)
4. Cool-down: 2 minutes of Child's Pose

Tip: Increase difficulty by adding weights, explosive movements, or reducing rest time.

WORKOUT 33:

1. Warm-up: 1 minute of Dynamic Lunges
2. Circuit: Perform 40s work / 20s rest per exercise
- Jump Squats
- Squats
- Burpees
- Single-Leg Deadlifts (bodyweight)
- Russian Twists
3. Repeat circuit for 3 rounds (about 15 minutes total)
4. Cool-down: 2 minutes of Child's Pose

Tip: Increase difficulty by adding weights, explosive movements, or reducing rest time.

WORKOUT 34:

1. Warm-up: 1 minute of Jog in Place
2. Circuit: Perform 20s work / 10s rest per exercise
- Sumo Squats
- High Knees
- Dead Bugs
- Plank
- Lateral Bounds
3. Repeat circuit for 6 rounds (about 15 minutes total)
4. Cool-down: 2 minutes of Downward Dog

Tip: Increase difficulty by adding weights, explosive movements, or reducing rest time.

WORKOUT 35:

1. Warm-up: 1 minute of Jog in Place
2. Circuit: Perform 40s work / 20s rest per exercise
- Jump Squats
- Hollow Hold
- V-Ups
- Lunges
- Bird Dogs
3. Repeat circuit for 3 rounds (about 15 minutes total)
4. Cool-down: 2 minutes of Hip Flexor Stretch

Tip: Increase difficulty by adding weights, explosive movements, or reducing rest time.

WORKOUT 36:

1. Warm-up: 1 minute of Butt Kicks
2. Circuit: Perform 20s work / 10s rest per exercise
- Calf Raises
- Leg Raises
- Frog Jumps
- Push-ups
- Star Jumps
3. Repeat circuit for 6 rounds (about 15 minutes total)
4. Cool-down: 2 minutes of alternating quad stretch

Tip: Increase difficulty by adding weights, explosive movements, or reducing rest time.

WORKOUT 37:

1. Warm-up: 1 minute of inchworms
2. Circuit: Perform 40s work / 20s rest per exercise
- Single-Leg Deadlifts (bodyweight)
- Jump Rope
- Lateral Bounds
- Mountain Climbers
- Flutter Kicks
3. Repeat circuit for 3 rounds (about 15 minutes total)
4. Cool-down: 2 minutes of Seated Twist

Tip: Increase difficulty by adding weights, explosive movements, or reducing rest time.

WORKOUT 38:

1. Warm-up: 1 minute of High Knees (low intensity)
2. Circuit: Perform 20s work / 10s rest per exercise
- Hollow Hold
- Sumo Squats
- Jumping Lunges
- Glute Bridges
- V-Ups
3. Repeat circuit for 6 rounds (about 15 minutes total)
4. Cool-down: 2 minutes of Hamstring Stretch

Tip: Increase difficulty by adding weights, explosive movements, or reducing rest time.

WORKOUT 39:

1. Warm-up: 1 minute of High Knees (low intensity)
2. Circuit: Perform 40s work / 20s rest per exercise
- Hollow Hold
- Jump Rope
- Bird Dogs
- Frog Jumps
- Tricep Dips
3. Repeat circuit for 3 rounds (about 15 minutes total)
4. Cool-down: 2 minutes of Forward Fold Stretch

Tip: Increase difficulty by adding weights, explosive movements, or reducing rest time.

WORKOUT 40:

1. Warm-up: 1 minute of Shadow Boxing
2. Circuit: Perform 20s work / 10s rest per exercise
- High Knees
- Glute Bridges
- Sumo Squats
- Jump Squats
- Tricep Dips
3. Repeat circuit for 6 rounds (about 15 minutes total)
4. Cool-down: 2 minutes of Forward Fold Stretch

Tip: Increase difficulty by adding weights, explosive movements, or reducing rest time.

WORKOUT 41:

1. Warm-up: 1 minute of Shadow Boxing
2. Circuit: Perform 40s work / 20s rest per exercise
- Jump Rope
- Squats
- Leg Raises
- Side Plank
- V-Ups
3. Repeat circuit for 3 rounds (about 15 minutes total)
4. Cool-down: 2 minutes of alternating quad stretch

Tip: Increase difficulty by adding weights, explosive movements, or reducing rest time.

WORKOUT 42:

1. Warm-up: 1 minute of Dynamic Lunges
2. Circuit: Perform 20s work / 10s rest per exercise
- Burpees
- Jump Squats
- Bird Dogs
- Jump Rope
- Tricep Dips
3. Repeat circuit for 6 rounds (about 15 minutes total)
4. Cool-down: 2 minutes of alternating quad stretch

Tip: Increase difficulty by adding weights, explosive movements, or reducing rest time.

WORKOUT 43:

1. Warm-up: 1 minute of Shadow Boxing
2. Circuit: Perform 40s work / 20s rest per exercise
- Glute Bridges
- Star Jumps
- Tricep Dips
- Step-Ups
- Calf Raises
3. Repeat circuit for 3 rounds (about 15 minutes total)
4. Cool-down: 2 minutes of Downward Dog

Tip: Increase difficulty by adding weights, explosive movements, or reducing rest time.

WORKOUT 44:

1. Warm-up: 1 minute of High Knees (low intensity)
2. Circuit: Perform 20s work / 10s rest per exercise
- Jump Squats
- Leg Raises
- Single-Leg Deadlifts (bodyweight)
- Skater Jumps
- Calf Raises
3. Repeat circuit for 6 rounds (about 15 minutes total)
4. Cool-down: 2 minutes of Hamstring Stretch

Tip: Increase difficulty by adding weights, explosive movements, or reducing rest time.

WORKOUT 45:

1. Warm-up: 1 minute of High Knees (low intensity)
2. Circuit: Perform 40s work / 20s rest per exercise
- Side Plank
- Squats
- Lunges
- Bird Dogs
- Leg Raises
3. Repeat circuit for 3 rounds (about 15 minutes total)
4. Cool-down: 2 minutes of Child's Pose

Tip: Increase difficulty by adding weights, explosive movements, or reducing rest time.

WORKOUT 46:

1. Warm-up: 1 minute of Jog in Place
2. Circuit: Perform 20s work / 10s rest per exercise
- Tricep Dips
- Jumping Lunges
- Leg Raises
- High Knees
- Star Jumps
3. Repeat circuit for 6 rounds (about 15 minutes total)
4. Cool-down: 2 minutes of Forward Fold Stretch

Tip: Increase difficulty by adding weights, explosive movements, or reducing rest time.

WORKOUT 47:

1. Warm-up: 1 minute of High Knees (low intensity)
2. Circuit: Perform 40s work / 20s rest per exercise
- Bird Dogs
- Jump Rope
- Toe Touches
- Bicycle Crunches
- Russian Twists
3. Repeat circuit for 3 rounds (about 15 minutes total)
4. Cool-down: 2 minutes of Child's Pose

Tip: Increase difficulty by adding weights, explosive movements, or reducing rest time.

WORKOUT 48:

1. Warm-up: 1 minute of Dynamic Lunges
2. Circuit: Perform 20s work / 10s rest per exercise
- Hollow Hold
- Mountain Climbers
- Jump Squats
- Leg Raises
- Side Plank
3. Repeat circuit for 6 rounds (about 15 minutes total)
4. Cool-down: 2 minutes of Hip Flexor Stretch

Tip: Increase difficulty by adding weights, explosive movements, or reducing rest time.

WORKOUT 49:

1. Warm-up: 1 minute of Butt Kicks
2. Circuit: Perform 40s work / 20s rest per exercise
- Bird Dogs
- Lunges
- Jump Squats
- High Knees
- Star Jumps
3. Repeat circuit for 3 rounds (about 15 minutes total)
4. Cool-down: 2 minutes of Child's Pose

Tip: Increase difficulty by adding weights, explosive movements, or reducing rest time.

WORKOUT 50:

1. Warm-up: 1 minute of Jog in Place
2. Circuit: Perform 20s work / 10s rest per exercise
- Tricep Dips
- Bicycle Crunches
- Flutter Kicks
- Push-ups
- Russian Twists
3. Repeat circuit for 6 rounds (about 15 minutes total)
4. Cool-down: 2 minutes of Cat-Cow Stretch

Tip: Increase difficulty by adding weights, explosive movements, or reducing rest time.

WORKOUT 51:

1. Warm-up: 1 minute of inchworms
2. Circuit: Perform 40s work / 20s rest per exercise
- Single-Leg Deadlifts (bodyweight)
- High Knees
- V-Ups
- Tricep Dips
- Calf Raises
3. Repeat circuit for 3 rounds (about 15 minutes total)
4. Cool-down: 2 minutes of Hip Flexor Stretch

Tip: Increase difficulty by adding weights, explosive movements, or reducing rest time.

WORKOUT 52:

1. Warm-up: 1 minute of Jumping Jacks
2. Circuit: Perform 20s work / 10s rest per exercise
- V-Ups
- Skater Jumps
- Glute Bridges
- Russian Twists
- Jump Rope
3. Repeat circuit for 6 rounds (about 15 minutes total)
4. Cool-down: 2 minutes of Cat-Cow Stretch

Tip: Increase difficulty by adding weights, explosive movements, or reducing rest time.

WORKOUT 53:

1. Warm-up: 1 minute of Shadow Boxing
2. Circuit: Perform 40s work / 20s rest per exercise
- V-Ups
- Step-Ups
- Bird Dogs
- Lateral Bounds
- Mountain Climbers
3. Repeat circuit for 3 rounds (about 15 minutes total)
4. Cool-down: 2 minutes of Seated Twist

Tip: Increase difficulty by adding weights, explosive movements, or reducing rest time.

WORKOUT 54:

1. Warm-up: 1 minute of Butt Kicks
2. Circuit: Perform 20s work / 10s rest per exercise
- Dead Bugs
- Toe Touches
- Plank
- Skater Jumps
- Calf Raises
3. Repeat circuit for 6 rounds (about 15 minutes total)
4. Cool-down: 2 minutes of Forward Fold Stretch

Tip: Increase difficulty by adding weights, explosive movements, or reducing rest time.

WORKOUT 55:

1. Warm-up: 1 minute of Arm Circles
2. Circuit: Perform 40s work / 20s rest per exercise
- Hollow Hold
- Plank
- Leg Raises
- Jump Rope
- Push-ups
3. Repeat circuit for 3 rounds (about 15 minutes total)
4. Cool-down: 2 minutes of Hip Flexor Stretch

Tip: Increase difficulty by adding weights, explosive movements, or reducing rest time.

WORKOUT 56:

1. Warm-up: 1 minute of Side Shuffles
2. Circuit: Perform 20s work / 10s rest per exercise
- Dead Bugs
- Jumping Lunges
- Sprint in Place
- Side Plank
- Flutter Kicks
3. Repeat circuit for 6 rounds (about 15 minutes total)
4. Cool-down: 2 minutes of Forward Fold Stretch

Tip: Increase difficulty by adding weights, explosive movements, or reducing rest time.

WORKOUT 57:

1. Warm-up: 1 minute of Jumping Jacks
2. Circuit: Perform 40s work / 20s rest per exercise
- Frog Jumps
- Glute Bridges
- Toe Touches
- Russian Twists
- Jumping Lunges
3. Repeat circuit for 3 rounds (about 15 minutes total)
4. Cool-down: 2 minutes of Cat-Cow Stretch

Tip: Increase difficulty by adding weights, explosive movements, or reducing rest time.

WORKOUT 58:

1. Warm-up: 1 minute of Side Shuffles
2. Circuit: Perform 20s work / 10s rest per exercise
- High Knees
- Leg Raises
- Mountain Climbers (slow)
- Star Jumps
- Sprint in Place
3. Repeat circuit for 6 rounds (about 15 minutes total)
4. Cool-down: 2 minutes of Seated Twist

Tip: Increase difficulty by adding weights, explosive movements, or reducing rest time.

WORKOUT 59:

1. Warm-up: 1 minute of Dynamic Lunges
2. Circuit: Perform 40s work / 20s rest per exercise
- High Knees
- Side Plank
- Squats
- Mountain Climbers (slow)
- Glute Bridges
3. Repeat circuit for 3 rounds (about 15 minutes total)
4. Cool-down: 2 minutes of Hamstring Stretch

Tip: Increase difficulty by adding weights, explosive movements, or reducing rest time.

WORKOUT 60:

1. Warm-up: 1 minute of Shadow Boxing
2. Circuit: Perform 20s work / 10s rest per exercise
- Dead Bugs
- Jump Rope
- Burpees
- Russian Twists
- Pike Push-ups
3. Repeat circuit for 6 rounds (about 15 minutes total)
4. Cool-down: 2 minutes of Hip Flexor Stretch

Tip: Increase difficulty by adding weights, explosive movements, or reducing rest time.

WORKOUT 61:

1. Warm-up: 1 minute of Shadow Boxing
2. Circuit: Perform 40s work / 20s rest per exercise
- Mountain Climbers
- Toe Touches
- Jump Squats
- Lateral Bounds
- Side Plank
3. Repeat circuit for 3 rounds (about 15 minutes total)
4. Cool-down: 2 minutes of Cat-Cow Stretch

Tip: Increase difficulty by adding weights, explosive movements, or reducing rest time.

WORKOUT 62:

1. Warm-up: 1 minute of Jumping Jacks
2. Circuit: Perform 20s work / 10s rest per exercise
- Dead Bugs
- Star Jumps
- Sumo Squats
- Hollow Hold
- Leg Raises
3. Repeat circuit for 6 rounds (about 15 minutes total)
4. Cool-down: 2 minutes of Forward Fold Stretch

Tip: Increase difficulty by adding weights, explosive movements, or reducing rest time.

WORKOUT 63:

1. Warm-up: 1 minute of Jumping Jacks
2. Circuit: Perform 40s work / 20s rest per exercise
- Mountain Climbers (slow)
- Sumo Squats
- Frog Jumps
- Single-Leg Deadlifts (bodyweight)
- Tricep Dips
3. Repeat circuit for 3 rounds (about 15 minutes total)
4. Cool-down: 2 minutes of alternating quad stretch

Tip: Increase difficulty by adding weights, explosive movements, or reducing rest time.

WORKOUT 64:

1. Warm-up: 1 minute of Jumping Jacks
2. Circuit: Perform 20s work / 10s rest per exercise
- Skater Jumps
- Mountain Climbers
- Dead Bugs
- Sumo Squats
- High Knees
3. Repeat circuit for 6 rounds (about 15 minutes total)
4. Cool-down: 2 minutes of Hip Flexor Stretch

Tip: Increase difficulty by adding weights, explosive movements, or reducing rest time.

WORKOUT 65:

1. Warm-up: 1 minute of Side Shuffles
2. Circuit: Perform 40s work / 20s rest per exercise
- Hollow Hold
- Burpees
- Frog Jumps
- Sumo Squats
- Jumping Lunges
3. Repeat circuit for 3 rounds (about 15 minutes total)
4. Cool-down: 2 minutes of Forward Fold Stretch

Tip: Increase difficulty by adding weights, explosive movements, or reducing rest time.

WORKOUT 66:

1. Warm-up: 1 minute of Jumping Jacks
2. Circuit: Perform 20s work / 10s rest per exercise
- Hollow Hold
- Mountain Climbers
- Bird Dogs
- Squats
- Pike Push-ups
3. Repeat circuit for 6 rounds (about 15 minutes total)
4. Cool-down: 2 minutes of alternating quad stretch

Tip: Increase difficulty by adding weights, explosive movements, or reducing rest time.

WORKOUT 67:

1. Warm-up: 1 minute of Side Shuffles
2. Circuit: Perform 40s work / 20s rest per exercise
- Skater Jumps
- High Knees
- Single-Leg Deadlifts (bodyweight)
- Push-ups
- V-Ups
3. Repeat circuit for 3 rounds (about 15 minutes total)
4. Cool-down: 2 minutes of Child's Pose

Tip: Increase difficulty by adding weights, explosive movements, or reducing rest time.

WORKOUT 68:

1. Warm-up: 1 minute of Shadow Boxing
2. Circuit: Perform 20s work / 10s rest per exercise
- Push-ups
- Bicycle Crunches
- Pike Push-ups
- Toe Touches
- Russian Twists
3. Repeat circuit for 6 rounds (about 15 minutes total)
4. Cool-down: 2 minutes of Downward Dog

Tip: Increase difficulty by adding weights, explosive movements, or reducing rest time.

WORKOUT 69:

1. Warm-up: 1 minute of Arm Circles
2. Circuit: Perform 40s work / 20s rest per exercise
- Mountain Climbers (slow)
- Bicycle Crunches
- Toe Touches
- Leg Raises
- Push-ups
3. Repeat circuit for 3 rounds (about 15 minutes total)
4. Cool-down: 2 minutes of Forward Fold Stretch

Tip: Increase difficulty by adding weights, explosive movements, or reducing rest time.

WORKOUT 70:

1. Warm-up: 1 minute of Side Shuffles
2. Circuit: Perform 20s work / 10s rest per exercise
- Plank
- Tricep Dips
- Leg Raises
- Glute Bridges
- Pike Push-ups
3. Repeat circuit for 6 rounds (about 15 minutes total)
4. Cool-down: 2 minutes of Seated Twist

Tip: Increase difficulty by adding weights, explosive movements, or reducing rest time.

WORKOUT 71:

1. Warm-up: 1 minute of inchworms
2. Circuit: Perform 40s work / 20s rest per exercise
- Frog Jumps
- Hollow Hold
- Jump Squats
- Glute Bridges
- Plank
3. Repeat circuit for 3 rounds (about 15 minutes total)
4. Cool-down: 2 minutes of Downward Dog

Tip: Increase difficulty by adding weights, explosive movements, or reducing rest time.

WORKOUT 72:

1. Warm-up: 1 minute of Butt Kicks
2. Circuit: Perform 20s work / 10s rest per exercise
- Russian Twists
- Flutter Kicks
- V-Ups
- Calf Raises
- Lateral Bounds
3. Repeat circuit for 6 rounds (about 15 minutes total)
4. Cool-down: 2 minutes of Hamstring Stretch

Tip: Increase difficulty by adding weights, explosive movements, or reducing rest time.

WORKOUT 73:

1. Warm-up: 1 minute of inchworms
2. Circuit: Perform 40s work / 20s rest per exercise
- Leg Raises
- Frog Jumps
- Plank
- Bird Dogs
- Single-Leg Deadlifts (bodyweight)
3. Repeat circuit for 3 rounds (about 15 minutes total)
4. Cool-down: 2 minutes of alternating quad stretch

Tip: Increase difficulty by adding weights, explosive movements, or reducing rest time.

WORKOUT 74:

1. Warm-up: 1 minute of Butt Kicks
2. Circuit: Perform 20s work / 10s rest per exercise
- Plank
- Step-Ups
- Burpees
- Mountain Climbers
- Squats
3. Repeat circuit for 6 rounds (about 15 minutes total)
4. Cool-down: 2 minutes of Cat-Cow Stretch

Tip: Increase difficulty by adding weights, explosive movements, or reducing rest time.

WORKOUT 75:

1. Warm-up: 1 minute of Jog in Place
2. Circuit: Perform 40s work / 20s rest per exercise
- Calf Raises
- Bicycle Crunches
- Push-ups
- Sprint in Place
- High Knees
3. Repeat circuit for 3 rounds (about 15 minutes total)
4. Cool-down: 2 minutes of Hamstring Stretch

Tip: Increase difficulty by adding weights, explosive movements, or reducing rest time.

WORKOUT 76:

1. Warm-up: 1 minute of Arm Circles
2. Circuit: Perform 20s work / 10s rest per exercise
- Sprint in Place
- Jump Squats
- Leg Raises
- Mountain Climbers
- V-Ups
3. Repeat circuit for 6 rounds (about 15 minutes total)
4. Cool-down: 2 minutes of Hip Flexor Stretch

Tip: Increase difficulty by adding weights, explosive movements, or reducing rest time.

WORKOUT 77:

1. Warm-up: 1 minute of Shadow Boxing
2. Circuit: Perform 40s work / 20s rest per exercise
- Side Plank
- Star Jumps
- Jump Squats
- Toe Touches
- Squats
3. Repeat circuit for 3 rounds (about 15 minutes total)
4. Cool-down: 2 minutes of Hip Flexor Stretch

Tip: Increase difficulty by adding weights, explosive movements, or reducing rest time.

WORKOUT 78:

1. Warm-up: 1 minute of Dynamic Lunges
2. Circuit: Perform 20s work / 10s rest per exercise
- Jumping Lunges
- Tricep Dips
- Skater Jumps
- Jump Squats
- Jump Rope
3. Repeat circuit for 6 rounds (about 15 minutes total)
4. Cool-down: 2 minutes of Hamstring Stretch

Tip: Increase difficulty by adding weights, explosive movements, or reducing rest time.

WORKOUT 79:

1. Warm-up: 1 minute of Side Shuffles
2. Circuit: Perform 40s work / 20s rest per exercise
- Single-Leg Deadlifts (bodyweight)
- Skater Jumps
- High Knees
- Lunges
- V-Ups
3. Repeat circuit for 3 rounds (about 15 minutes total)
4. Cool-down: 2 minutes of Seated Twist

Tip: Increase difficulty by adding weights, explosive movements, or reducing rest time.

WORKOUT 80:

1. Warm-up: 1 minute of Side Shuffles
2. Circuit: Perform 20s work / 10s rest per exercise
- Bicycle Crunches
- Squats
- Sprint in Place
- Sumo Squats
- Lunges
3. Repeat circuit for 6 rounds (about 15 minutes total)
4. Cool-down: 2 minutes of alternating quad stretch

Tip: Increase difficulty by adding weights, explosive movements, or reducing rest time.

WORKOUT 81:

1. Warm-up: 1 minute of Arm Circles
2. Circuit: Perform 40s work / 20s rest per exercise
- Sumo Squats
- Skater Jumps
- Star Jumps
- Push-ups
- Plank
3. Repeat circuit for 3 rounds (about 15 minutes total)
4. Cool-down: 2 minutes of Seated Twist

Tip: Increase difficulty by adding weights, explosive movements, or reducing rest time.

WORKOUT 82:

1. Warm-up: 1 minute of High Knees (low intensity)
2. Circuit: Perform 20s work / 10s rest per exercise
- Pike Push-ups
- Bicycle Crunches
- Bird Dogs
- Star Jumps
- Jump Rope
3. Repeat circuit for 6 rounds (about 15 minutes total)
4. Cool-down: 2 minutes of Cat-Cow Stretch

Tip: Increase difficulty by adding weights, explosive movements, or reducing rest time.

WORKOUT 83:

1. Warm-up: 1 minute of Butt Kicks
2. Circuit: Perform 40s work / 20s rest per exercise
- Star Jumps
- Plank
- Jump Squats
- V-Ups
- Frog Jumps
3. Repeat circuit for 3 rounds (about 15 minutes total)
4. Cool-down: 2 minutes of Seated Twist

Tip: Increase difficulty by adding weights, explosive movements, or reducing rest time.

WORKOUT 84:

1. Warm-up: 1 minute of inchworms
2. Circuit: Perform 20s work / 10s rest per exercise
- Skater Jumps
- Burpees
- Glute Bridges
- Plank
- Lunges
3. Repeat circuit for 6 rounds (about 15 minutes total)
4. Cool-down: 2 minutes of Seated Twist

Tip: Increase difficulty by adding weights, explosive movements, or reducing rest time.

WORKOUT 85:

1. Warm-up: 1 minute of Jumping Jacks
2. Circuit: Perform 40s work / 20s rest per exercise
- Tricep Dips
- Flutter Kicks
- Burpees
- Hollow Hold
- Lunges
3. Repeat circuit for 3 rounds (about 15 minutes total)
4. Cool-down: 2 minutes of Hamstring Stretch

Tip: Increase difficulty by adding weights, explosive movements, or reducing rest time.

WORKOUT 86:

1. Warm-up: 1 minute of High Knees (low intensity)
2. Circuit: Perform 20s work / 10s rest per exercise
- Frog Jumps
- Jump Rope
- Lunges
- Calf Raises
- Hollow Hold
3. Repeat circuit for 6 rounds (about 15 minutes total)
4. Cool-down: 2 minutes of Cat-Cow Stretch

Tip: Increase difficulty by adding weights, explosive movements, or reducing rest time.

WORKOUT 87:

1. Warm-up: 1 minute of High Knees (low intensity)
2. Circuit: Perform 40s work / 20s rest per exercise
- Single-Leg Deadlifts (bodyweight)
- Star Jumps
- Jumping Lunges
- Lateral Bounds
- Mountain Climbers
3. Repeat circuit for 3 rounds (about 15 minutes total)
4. Cool-down: 2 minutes of Hip Flexor Stretch

Tip: Increase difficulty by adding weights, explosive movements, or reducing rest time.

WORKOUT 88:

1. Warm-up: 1 minute of Butt Kicks
2. Circuit: Perform 20s work / 10s rest per exercise
- Mountain Climbers
- Dead Bugs
- Step-Ups
- Sumo Squats
- V-Ups
3. Repeat circuit for 6 rounds (about 15 minutes total)
4. Cool-down: 2 minutes of Hip Flexor Stretch

Tip: Increase difficulty by adding weights, explosive movements, or reducing rest time.

WORKOUT 89:

1. Warm-up: 1 minute of Arm Circles
2. Circuit: Perform 40s work / 20s rest per exercise
- Tricep Dips
- Step-Ups
- Plank
- Jump Squats
- V-Ups
3. Repeat circuit for 3 rounds (about 15 minutes total)
4. Cool-down: 2 minutes of Cat-Cow Stretch

Tip: Increase difficulty by adding weights, explosive movements, or reducing rest time.

WORKOUT 90:

1. Warm-up: 1 minute of Jog in Place
2. Circuit: Perform 20s work / 10s rest per exercise
- Lateral Bounds
- High Knees
- Hollow Hold
- Burpees
- Bird Dogs
3. Repeat circuit for 6 rounds (about 15 minutes total)
4. Cool-down: 2 minutes of Cat-Cow Stretch

Tip: Increase difficulty by adding weights, explosive movements, or reducing rest time.

WORKOUT 91:

1. Warm-up: 1 minute of Jog in Place
2. Circuit: Perform 40s work / 20s rest per exercise
- Jumping Lunges
- Lateral Bounds
- Mountain Climbers (slow)
- Bird Dogs
- Jump Squats
3. Repeat circuit for 3 rounds (about 15 minutes total)
4. Cool-down: 2 minutes of Seated Twist

Tip: Increase difficulty by adding weights, explosive movements, or reducing rest time.

WORKOUT 92:

1. Warm-up: 1 minute of inchworms
2. Circuit: Perform 20s work / 10s rest per exercise
- Russian Twists
- V-Ups
- Mountain Climbers
- Tricep Dips
- Dead Bugs
3. Repeat circuit for 6 rounds (about 15 minutes total)
4. Cool-down: 2 minutes of alternating quad stretch

Tip: Increase difficulty by adding weights, explosive movements, or reducing rest time.

WORKOUT 93:

1. Warm-up: 1 minute of inchworms
2. Circuit: Perform 40s work / 20s rest per exercise
- High Knees
- Squats
- Single-Leg Deadlifts (bodyweight)
- Sprint in Place
- Tricep Dips
3. Repeat circuit for 3 rounds (about 15 minutes total)
4. Cool-down: 2 minutes of Seated Twist

Tip: Increase difficulty by adding weights, explosive movements, or reducing rest time.

WORKOUT 94:

1. Warm-up: 1 minute of Arm Circles
2. Circuit: Perform 20s work / 10s rest per exercise
- Single-Leg Deadlifts (bodyweight)
- Leg Raises
- Side Plank
- Star Jumps
- Toe Touches
3. Repeat circuit for 6 rounds (about 15 minutes total)
4. Cool-down: 2 minutes of Forward Fold Stretch

Tip: Increase difficulty by adding weights, explosive movements, or reducing rest time.

WORKOUT 95:

1. Warm-up: 1 minute of Jog in Place
2. Circuit: Perform 40s work / 20s rest per exercise
- Squats
- V-Ups
- Calf Raises
- Glute Bridges
- Jump Rope
3. Repeat circuit for 3 rounds (about 15 minutes total)
4. Cool-down: 2 minutes of Child's Pose

Tip: Increase difficulty by adding weights, explosive movements, or reducing rest time.

WORKOUT 96:

1. Warm-up: 1 minute of Jog in Place
2. Circuit: Perform 20s work / 10s rest per exercise
- V-Ups
- Frog Jumps
- Mountain Climbers (slow)
- Step-Ups
- Jumping Lunges
3. Repeat circuit for 6 rounds (about 15 minutes total)
4. Cool-down: 2 minutes of alternating quad stretch

Tip: Increase difficulty by adding weights, explosive movements, or reducing rest time.

WORKOUT 97:

1. Warm-up: 1 minute of Dynamic Lunges
2. Circuit: Perform 40s work / 20s rest per exercise
- Bird Dogs
- Single-Leg Deadlifts (bodyweight)
- Plank
- Star Jumps
- High Knees
3. Repeat circuit for 3 rounds (about 15 minutes total)
4. Cool-down: 2 minutes of Child's Pose

Tip: Increase difficulty by adding weights, explosive movements, or reducing rest time.

WORKOUT 98:

1. Warm-up: 1 minute of Jumping Jacks
2. Circuit: Perform 20s work / 10s rest per exercise
- Jumping Lunges
- Pike Push-ups
- Star Jumps
- Skater Jumps
- Sumo Squats
3. Repeat circuit for 6 rounds (about 15 minutes total)
4. Cool-down: 2 minutes of Downward Dog

Tip: Increase difficulty by adding weights, explosive movements, or reducing rest time.

WORKOUT 99:

1. Warm-up: 1 minute of Shadow Boxing
2. Circuit: Perform 40s work / 20s rest per exercise
- Squats
- Flutter Kicks
- Toe Touches
- Skater Jumps
- V-Ups
3. Repeat circuit for 3 rounds (about 15 minutes total)
4. Cool-down: 2 minutes of alternating quad stretch

Tip: Increase difficulty by adding weights, explosive movements, or reducing rest time.

WORKOUT 100:

1. Warm-up: 1 minute of Arm Circles
2. Circuit: Perform 20s work / 10s rest per exercise
- Jumping Lunges
- Bird Dogs
- Side Plank
- Calf Raises
- Sprint in Place
3. Repeat circuit for 6 rounds (about 15 minutes total)
4. Cool-down: 2 minutes of Cat-Cow Stretch

Tip: Increase difficulty by adding weights, explosive movements, or reducing rest time.

WORKOUT 101:

1. Warm-up: 1 minute of Butt Kicks
2. Circuit: Perform 40s work / 20s rest per exercise
- Dead Bugs
- Burpees
- Leg Raises
- V-Ups
- Step-Ups
3. Repeat circuit for 3 rounds (about 15 minutes total)
4. Cool-down: 2 minutes of Hip Flexor Stretch

Tip: Increase difficulty by adding weights, explosive movements, or reducing rest time.

Printed in Dunstable, United Kingdom